Ask Maggie Rose

MANAGING LIFE'S SWEET SORROW

BY
MAGGIE ROSE

Introduction

Our better angels are those who can transform crisis, tragedy, and even death into moments and gifts that bring joy and life to those who remain. This is why I have always admired transplant teams, organ donors, and donors' generous families. They bring joy and life born out of their tragedies to those who remain. As a transplant recipient (corneal transplant), I have enjoyed much improved eyesight for a number of years; I know firsthand the joyous gifts of better angels.

I say this by way of introducing you to one of my own better angels, Maggie Rose. I first met this remarkable woman nearly a decade ago when I worked for her in a sales position with a large national consulting firm. I wasn't much of a salesman, and she knew that, but she gave me a chance at a time when I needed a chance. I didn't last long with that company, but our friendship has remained solid ever since.

In my darkest hours, I reached out for the hand of a friend, and it was Maggie Rose's hand that was there for me. She dropped everything she was doing and rushed to my side. She held me up and loved me through a dark valley. On the other side, I emerged to a new life that eventually included attaining my masters in social work and a doctorate in the same field. Today, I teach social work at a state university.

Students benefit from my life's experiences and my education. They don't know that they have Maggie Rose to thank for those gifts as much as anyone. She was the "transplant doctor" that brought about this change.

Here, in these few brief pages, you are going to meet people from all walks of life. Each has taken on the care of an aging parent or spouse. Each is reaching out in the darkness for help, for wisdom, or for courage. The hand they touch is Maggie Rose's hand. She shares her wondrous wisdom and her remarkable courage with each of them – and now with me and with you. Her thoughts come not from a textbook but from the hard school of life. You will hear the story of her own mother's stroke. You will learn how love and forgiveness and second chances can change our destinies, as Maggie Rose changed hers and her mother's destinies.

Above all else, you are about to meet a friend. One of the real joys of my life has always been sharing friends – that delicious moment when you introduce one friend to another, knowing that both of their lives are about to be greatly enhanced by the synergies of new friendships forged. In this short introduction, I have the great pleasure to introduce you to a new friend – one of my oldest and dearest friends – the inimitable, indefatigable Maggie Rose.

David H. Johnson, Ph.D.
Millersville, Pennsylvania
June 13, 2011

Forward

It is a delight knowing that the community and now, caregivers all over will have the benefit of enjoying Maggie Rose's wisdom in this bound collection of her *Citizen-Herald* columns. The idea for "Ask Maggie Rose" came about in 2007, after the Council on Aging learned that the current long term and popular senior opinion page was being cancelled due to a new policy by the paper stating that syndicated columns by writers in other communities could no longer be published. After initially feeling disappointed by this news, I recalled that one of our family caregivers, Maggie Rose, who gave helpful advice to others was also a writer. I decided to approach her to see if she had any interest in writing a column on the subject of care giving. She bravely accepted and generously gave of her time and heart to the many family members who posed challenging and intimate questions about their experiences. It has now been three years of people sending in poignant stories of their struggles and conflicts in caring for their elder loved ones. Maggie Rose gives voice to and affirms the dignity of their unique struggles, in effect, lightening their burdens and breaking the isolation and loneliness that are the hallmark of the care giving experience. She evaluates their ethical dilemmas non-judgmentally, yet the clear direction she provides them is moral in the best sense. Whatever situation is presented to her, she always, *always,* communicates back to her readers with great warmth and empathy. Family members in all stages in the life cycle will find these pieces, as well as her poetry and prose, enriching.

Nava Niv-Vogel LICSW, M.P.H
Director of Belmont Council on Aging

"For in all the world there are no people so...forlorn as those who are forced to eat the bitter bread of dependency in their old age, and find how steep are the stairs of another man's house..."
Dorothy Dix

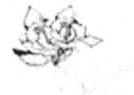

Dedication

I dedicate this book to the many, many seniors who do not have adequate resources to pay for long-term care and find that they must rely on family and friends to care for them, and to the more than sixty-five-million family members or friends who provide that care. According to the National Alliance for Caregiving in collaboration with AARP; November 2009, "... 29% of the U.S. population provide care for a chronically ill, disabled, or aged family member or friend during any given year." Adult caregivers don't just give a few minutes out of their day providing care for a loved one; for most, they spend twenty or more hours a week, and for many, caregiving is a full-time second job. In a similar report, *Young Caregivers in the U.S. 2005, the National Alliance for Caregiving and the United Hospital Fund* state that 1.4 million children ages 8 to 18 provide care for an adult relative; 72% are caring for a parent or grandparent; and 64% live in the same household as their care recipient.

A recent study from AARP estimates that family caregivers deliver $450 billion in care to their loved ones each year. That is almost as much as America spends on Medicare, and it is nearly four times what Medicaid spends on long-term care.

And

I dedicate this book in loving memory of my Mother. She is the beautiful woman you see on the cover.

Marjorie Cantwell

9-26-1928 ~ 3-06-2009

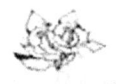

"There is no way to talk about that exact moment when you re-alize the certainty of an impending loss without sounding trite and self-pitying. All of it has been said before and in thousands of different ways, but the importance of those first and sometimes-final seconds before calamity claims someone we love there is a naked honesty that has a simple and pure quality to it where we can once again discover unconditional love and the joy of selflessness. Life's most important moments are the ones we share that are basked in the tenderness of that selflessness."

Maggie Rose

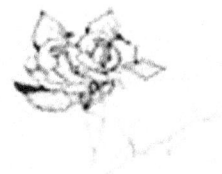

The Simple Moments

I can never forget the night my mother had her stroke; it was Tuesday, January 25, 2006. I was at home in Conyers, Georgia, when Alice, my youngest sister, called. The call came at seven-thirty that evening. My family was just finishing dinner. I checked the caller ID—such a twentieth-century thing to do—and saw it was Alice calling from Belmont, Massachusetts. I could not remember the last time that she had called during the week! Alarmed, I grabbed the phone. "Mom is in the hospital." Alice's voice shook. I barely recognized her. "No one can talk to her; we need someone from the family to go to Panama City, Florida, right away!"

Our mother had been vacationing in Florida alone, something she had started to do regularly since she realized that John, her husband, would not retire. I made Alice repeat what she had just said. I was having trouble believing what she was saying. I struggled for coherency. Then I asked, "Where is John?"

Never would I have guessed what she told me next. Earlier that day John's retina had detached from his cornea, and he was in Massachusetts General Hospital. As Alice and I were speaking, our stepfather was waiting for emergency surgery to save his eyesight.

1

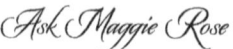

Their marriage, like Mama's life, had always had a lot of division. At approximately the same time that day, each of them had suffered their separate emergencies: she in Florida and he in Massachusetts. I guess it was fitting that circumstances would force them apart at this critical time in life. Mama always felt that God had an odd sense of humor.

Only on a soap opera could you expect such drama, but this was real life. After the surgery, John would not be able to fly or drive until he was released from his surgeon's care. That would be months. Since my husband and I lived in Georgia, it made sense for me to fly to Florida. I booked my reservation for the first flight out in the morning: a 5:45 a.m. departure. I packed only a small overnight bag. Who knows what I was thinking?

Mother was a single-minded woman, and no one could have stopped her from going to Florida alone. I had never tried to stop her. For eight years she had been taking this annual trip, but this time I had had some sense of dread when I left her in Florida just a few short weeks past. Panama City Beach was where she liked to vacation. She had many friends, all fellow snowbirds who vacationed in the same complex. Still, I was uncomfortable leaving her. I had had the feeling that I may never see her again, and I had cried most of the way home after I left her. In some ways, she had become like a child to me: wanting, expecting, insisting, and unable to distinguish the boundaries of what would be safe. She did not know her limits.

I knew she was lonesome for John and for family, but this choice to go to Florida alone was hers and she was going to stand by it. She had many medical diagnoses that indicated there could be a problem, but our mother was not a woman to live in fear of anything. She was a woman who lived.

Over the last decade, she had made several trips to various spots all over the southeastern United States: the Houston Space Center; the site of the Alamo in Austin, Texas; a trip to Warm Springs and Calloway Gardens in Georgia; the Kennedy Space Center; a little gambling in Biloxi, Mississippi. The list went on. She had also been on two different cruises: one to the western Caribbean and one to Mexico. She had explored Panama City, Florida, fully. She had many pictures framed and displayed around her vacation condominium in Sunny Side, Florida. She also had many of the photos copied and displayed at her beach home on Cape Cod and her permanent residence in Belmont, Massachusetts. They served as a reminder to all of us that she was having fun.

My attention, no longer on the phone call I had just received from Alice, wandered to a mental image of her hurt and alone. It pained me to think of her alone in a hospital. Her fun was over.

I called the hospital several times during that evening, but I got the same answers every time. "Mrs. Cantwell is in the emergency room; she is unable to come to the phone. She is in critical condition."

"Why can't you bring the phone to her?" I asked with trepidation.

"She is unable to speak at this time."

That was it! They would give no more information until someone presented them with proof of a health proxy or power of attorney. Both were in her purse, but the hospital staff was unable to find either one. From their answers, I guessed that she had had a stroke. What other possible explanation could there be to explain why she could not come to the phone?

I went to bed late that night, and I did not fall asleep until a few minutes before the alarm went off. I arrived at the airport much too

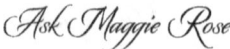

early, barely coherent, and alone. I called the hospital one last time before I boarded my plane. This time when they told me that she was still in the emergency room, I lost all control. I screamed into the phone. "Why isn't she in a room? Why is she still in emergency? Why can't I talk to her? If my mother is dead, tell me now! Tell—me—now!"

"No, Miss March,"—in the South, everyone is Miss—"she is not dead." I swear I heard her start to say *yet*. "But please get here as soon as you can." The nurse was earnest, and I believed her, but I also believe she had purposefully left off the *yet*.

It is only a one-hour flight from Atlanta to Panama City. It felt like ten. The cab ride from Panama City Airport to the hospital was short. The driver was silent; obviously, he had made this trip to the hospital before. When I paid him, he offered me his card and asked me where I was going when I left the hospital. I told him my mother rented in Sunny Side (a quiet spot at the west end of the beach) and explained that I would call for a cab when I was ready to leave. He advised me that it might be difficult to find anyone to go as far west as I would need to go to get to my mother's condominium. He wrote his home number on the back of his card and offered to come back if I had a problem, and he told me to call at any hour—I was amazed that a cabdriver would be so thoughtful. His name was Binky; you do not forget a name like that.

I stepped outside the cab, and the sounds of morning were determined, urgent, and incessant. The air was salty, and sea gulls screeched overhead. As I turned, I felt a warm, gentle breeze caress my face. The scent of the ocean, a familiar friend, relaxed me. I closed my eyes and took a slow, deep breath, and as I exhaled, I let the comfort of Florida's winter sun warm me. Crickets! Birds! Cars! Suddenly, the day was alive! It was hard for me to believe what I knew I was going to face. I took another slow, deep breath. I placed one foot deliberately in front of the other, and with firm, steady strides, I followed the signs that read "Emergency Room."

The automatic doors parted as I entered. I met with no resistance; doctors, nurses, aides, security, everybody moved out of my way. My instincts led the way; then I saw her purse—we had shopped for it together. It was visible from under the hospital's dreary green curtain. I knew she was "behind curtain number one!" I remember thinking, "What an absurd thing to think!" I quietly pulled the curtain aside. My hand shook. She saw me immediately. Our eyes locked. I froze. It took a minute for me to realize that the throbbing in my ears was my heart.

We had been here before, Mama and me: her lying amid white linens and gauze, ashen and on the verge of death. However, I had never seen her quite so frail, and never had her face been so twisted or her body so obviously assaulted. Looking at her, I felt certain she must of have had a stroke. Maybe it was because we had always been so close that we spoke so honestly and with so few words. I could not speak much. Pain held my throat with vicious intent as if to warn of what was to come. Our eyes stayed fixed on each other as the moment preyed upon us. She was alive, barely, but alive!

"Hi, my little Rosy Nose." Her words were barely audible, but her eyes smiled; the fire was still there. She lifted her weakened right arm, and with her fingertip, she tapped my nose as I leaned in toward her. The left side of her face drooped. The mouth—not quite like a mouth anymore—paralyzed by the stroke, had caused the words to slur out of the right side of her lips. She spoke again. This time she spoke more distinctly. She pushed the words out of the twisted pucker at the right side of her face and said, "Don't faint!"

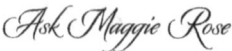

She was clearly my mother, half dead, but her concern was for me. Forty years earlier when I had seen her lying on an emergency room stretcher, the moment our eyes had met; I had fainted, so her motherly concern was justified.

Her words were still ringing in my ears. I wanted to speak. My mind was struggling for something to say, but before I could speak, the shift in her eyes showed her fear. "Mama," I said still fighting my tears. It was all that would come out. I went to her stretcher and lowered the metal sidebar. I placed my face against hers with my nose touching her right cheek and my left cheek on her pillow, I wrapped my right arm around her as tightly as I dared, feeling for the first time the listlessness of her left side. "I love you, Mama; I love you." I fought the tears for her sake, not for mine. Mama lay still, and for a few minutes we let the silence, the love, the seriousness of the present, dance over us.

Mama survived her stroke. It paralyzed her left side, and she suffered serious brain damage. She did not lose her memories or her ability to recognize her family, and she remembers everyone's name. She does sometimes confuse dreams with reality, but then she always did. She never forgets that things have happened, but she has trouble remembering the order of events and if they happened recently or a long while ago. She can still make value judgments for herself, but she has lost the desire to pass judgment on anyone or anything. The stroke has made her wiser, more loving, and humble. Those are all things you must hold on to in order to survive being an invalid. She is completely dependent.

Mama had her eightieth birthday in September 2008. We do not think she will have an eighty-first birthday. I have not forgotten those first few minutes I spent in the emergency room with her, nor have I lost the understanding of how precious each second of life is. I have learned a lot about love, and that love is not love until you give it away. At the same time, an even greater gift is to be able to accept love with graciousness and to delight in its simplicity.

There is no way to talk about that exact moment when you realize the certainty of an impending loss without sounding trite and self-pity-ing. All of it has been said before and in thousands of different ways, but the importance of those first and sometimes-final seconds before calamity claims someone we love there is a naked honesty that has a simple and pure quality to it, where we can once again discover un-conditional love and the joy of selflessness. Life's most important mo-ments are the ones we share that are basked in the tenderness of that selflessness.

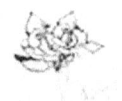

The Hush of Goodbye

I did not know you would be so still

Like the hush just before daybreak

Those moments when, if you

Should awake, you might be confused:

So deep in the night, so close to the day...

You, lost between two worlds

I did not know you would be so still

Like the mist quiet upon the snow

You cannot imagine that any footprints

Should tread there:

So deep in the moment, so close to the way...

Me, Lost between two worlds

I did not know you would be so still

Like a fire spent, no embers there

To stoke its ashes would only be senseless

Should fire burn:

So deep in the loss, so close to the grave...

You and me, between two worlds

Hush now, sleep my love...

I will be here, waiting no more.

Maggie Rose

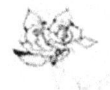

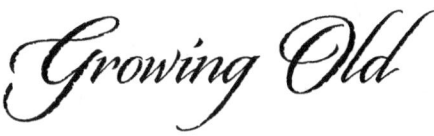

Growing Old

Dear Maggie Rose,

I really enjoyed meeting you at Judith's party. You are a gracious and funny woman. I hope we can get to know each other and become great friends.

I am anxious about my fast approaching sixtieth birthday. I wasn't fooling around when I said I was looking for ways to grow old gracefully. I don't think sixty is old; in fact, Judith looks so good I am starting to think that sixty is the new thirty. However, the natural forward progression of sixty leaves me quaking in my boots. I am not ready for the next decade. Do you have any of your sage advice to help me handle this?

Sincerely,
Mary T
Watertown

Dear Mary,

I truly enjoyed meeting you at Judith's sixtieth birthday party. She prepared a delicious buffet, and I thought it was a nice celebration.

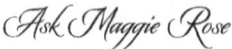

I agree with you that sixty is a monumental birthday, and I found it inspiring that Judith's health and appearance are so good. She looks terrific. I will forever be grateful to her for having the good sense to turn sixty before I did. She has certainly contradicted the conventional thinking concerning turning sixty. I don't agree with you that sixty is the new thirty, but perhaps it is the new fifty, and we should all be celebrating that. This brings me to the reason I write you today. You posed an interesting question at the party. I know because of my involvement at the senior center, that many of the ladies think of me as some type of expert concerning matters of aging. I assure you, I am not. All of my work is either self-serving or volunteer, although I am well studied, I have no credentials to back up any opinions that I might offer. Someone once told me that you should never give someone a piece of your mind without first stopping to consider if you can get by on what is left. That being said, I have thought long and hard about your query—"Tell me how to grow old gracefully?"

Mary, I am not sure if it can be done. The question, it seems to me, is an oxymoron. I have tried to think about an answer that would give us both some insights, something, simultaneously, brilliant and utilitarian. To be honest, I haven't found anything particularly graceful about growing older. As the adage goes: growing old is not for sissies. However, I did examine the meaning of the words that make up your question, and in those words, I found some comfort.

Let us start with the words "Tell me." Seeking advice from me is flattering; believe me, I am touched by your question. I would recommend, however, that it might be wiser to consult with someone who has expertise in the area of choice. You need someone who has already accomplished the desired results you're looking for. Mary, I'm just not old yet. I expect to be old someday. I say that only after considerable pondering of my alternative, but today I am still young.

How to do something, anything, starts with a basic desire to do. Doing is good. I think that anyone who embarks on a "how to" endeavor should become informed. There are many books available, all filled with pages and pages of information on the "how to" of every aspect of life, including growing old. I think some of these books are marvelous resources. I would caution you, however, not to get lost in this plethora of information. Life is about doing.

"Grow" is a marvelous word. I love to garden, to grow big beautiful roses along the fence at the back of my yard. I was one of those women who loved being pregnant. Feeling my child grow inside my womb was joyous. I thoroughly enjoy watching my grandchildren grow into the beautiful young people they are. Over the years, my interests have grown. My patience with others has grown. My tolerances of my differences with people have grown, and as time passes, my commitments have grown deeper. My love for my husband and family grows stronger daily. I realize that my days are growing shorter, and as they do, my memories grow fonder.

"Old," however, is not necessarily an inspiring word. We all love old houses; they have character and charm. We love old cities; they have history. We collect old coins; sometimes the older the coin the more value it has. Old furniture is so interesting to us we give it its own name, antiques. In fact, we do this for cars, jewelry, china, glassware, watches, sewing machines, washboards, dolls, weather vanes, and the list goes on. Moreover, if we find something really old, we give it a truly distinguished title; we call it a relic. Of course, when it comes to people, we simply call them old.

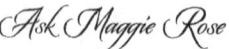

Old, when applied to people, doesn't conjure up any particularly exciting images, does it? Canes and walkers clacking down wide odorous hallways aren't the fodder of our hopes and dreams. Little old ladies counting out the exact change for their groceries, one nickel at a time, while we wait behind them, our patience growing thin, our eyes meeting others' with equal impatience, wondering how much more of our time will be frittered away during this tedious ritual, help us realize how much we value our time. Truly, in our society that covets instant food, instant pay, instant gratification, these doddering old folks are slowing us down. My point here, Mary, is that old is only good if you are not a person.

Grace is an eloquent word. It has many definitions and all of them touched by humility. Of course, grace can be spiritual, as in full of grace. This is about not just elegance or beauty of form, but a deep inner influence or spirit of God. There are also acts of grace: mercy, clemency, and pardon. We can have the grace to be kind to even the most disagreeable of foes during their time of great sorrow. Yes, I know that takes compassion, but isn't that the grace of moral strength, the grace to do what you know is right no matter how difficult the task? This elusive quest—to grow old gracefully—may not be attainable, but the choices we make can move us gracefully through life.

The only problematic word was old, and only when we used it with the word person. If we take "old" out of the question, we can ask, "How do we grow gracefully?" We don't have to do a thing about the old. If we are lucky, that cruel sweetness will happen all by itself. I think that what remains for us to do is to seek the most successful examples of people who have grown gracefully and emulate those inner qualities we find so desirous. As for me, I feel there is nothing more graceful than kindness, so it is with kindest intent that I offer you my humble advice and trust there are, at the very least, some elements of an answer.

I wish you and your family the very best.

Warmest Regards,
Maggie Rose

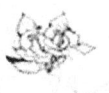

Feeling Pressured

Dear Maggie Rose,

I am the youngest of seven children. While growing up I was very close to my parents, and I still live within 7-miles of their home. I am a single mother with two children still at home, and I work a full time job. Because I live in close proximity to my parents, I have spent the most time with them.

Recently, my older sister who is 18 years my elder noticed that my father's mental health is not as crisp as it used to be. I do agree with her that he has shown some significant decline. That is not the problem. The problem is that she is telling my mother that I should move in with them so I can take care of them.

I love my parents dearly, but a move would be ridiculous. It would disrupt my children's school and social routines. I presently live less than a mile from my job. My mother is on top of the situation in her home. In time, a decision will have to be made. If my sister thinks it is so important that someone live with my parents, I think she and her husband should give up their home and take charge. Their children are long out of the nest.

My mother has not asked for my help, and I have not offered. Every time my sister calls my mother becomes anxious and agitated. I really think that these phone calls upset my mother. I don't remember my mother ever telling me she expected me to take care of her or my dad, and furthermore, we are not at that stage. How do I let my sister know that she needs to stop upsetting my mother and me? I honestly believe my mother can handle her own life right now.

Feeling pressured.

Dear Feeling Pressured,

Isn't family wonderful! Your sister's enthusiasm to pass the responsibility on to you and your children is comical, so try not to lose your sense of humor.

You did say that you noticed "...significant decline..." in your father's mental health. That is something that the family should stay on top of. Your mother might be hiding her concerns from you. I am sure she is dealing with many new challenges that the change in your dad's health has meant to her. Possibly, she does not want you to think she feels you should be responsible for their care. I want to be sure that you and your mother are clear that she does not have to handle your father's care alone. Many times, when we talk about caregivers, we forget how often the spouse is the primary caregiver.

After a lifetime of caring for each other, spouses are often reluctant to ask for help from their children or an outside agency. The expectations, responsibilities, and even the change in roles can be overwhelming. In your father's case, he has become the dependent instead of the provider. This would be unsettling to even the most stable of families.

My concern is not that you need to move in to provide support for your mother, but that your mother receives support from some source. I can promise you that a significant decline in mental health requires plenty of extra attention. I think your parents may be at "...that stage..." and that collectively, you and your siblings should make a family plan. The reason your mother may be so upset after your sister's phone calls might have something to do with her understanding the seriousness of the situation but not understanding where to turn for help.

I think it is important to point out that the behaviors you might observe on a visit are very different from the burdens of day-to-day care, and most likely, your mother is hiding that from you.

If your mother lives in Belmont, please refer her to our Council on Aging. If she lives in another town, then do the same for her in that town. Being a good daughter doesn't mean giving up your own life, but it does require that you take some initiative to ensure your parents' safety. There are many resources available to help our loved ones manage the inevitable challenges that aging can present. Our job is to help them find the best choices available. Your sister could assist by making some phone calls, on your mother's behalf, to the appropriate agencies. As I said, I do think the time has come for a good family plan. Please remember to take advantage of the services offered through the Council on Aging in your neighborhood.

I wish you and your family the best.

Warmest regards,
Maggie Rose

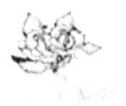

A Happy Teenager

Dear Maggie Rose,

I do not have a question as much as I want to say how happy I am that my grandmother has come to live with us. My mother thought it would be a good idea if I wrote you so other grandparents would know how nice it is to have them close and share family time with them. My grandmother really understands me, and unlike my parents, she never yells at me and she loves to help me with my English homework. She is teaching me how to knit and we have many laughs because my things never turn out as nicely as hers do, but I keep trying. Actually, the things she makes turn out to be sweaters, hats, slippers and such. The stuff I make turn out like things. My grandmother is the best, and I love having her live with us.

Sincerely,
A Happy Teenager

Dear Happy Teenager,

It was kind of you to share your story and I think others will benefit from it. I can tell from your letter that you and your grandmother are

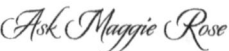

both blessed to have each other. Also, I want to thank your mother for the advice she gave to you. Whenever we reach out and have the courage to share some of the more private details of our daily lives, we help others, but just as importantly, it puts our feelings to the front of our own mind and we end up helping ourselves. I hope you feel proud of yourself and your family.

We always had extended family living with us. As a little girl, I lived in a big house near the ocean in Scituate, Massachusetts. Grammy (that is what we called my great-grandmother) was the center of my world. It's funny what a child will remember. I don't remember her face except for a vague visual imprint somewhere in the recesses of my mind. I do remember how, truly, she did love me. I can remember running to her every time my mother caught me doing some naughty little thing (a daily occurrence, I can assure you). Grammy would have no part of anyone scolding me for anything she thought was minor—and if I did it, it was minor—so my poor mother was hard pressed to delve out any discipline.

When Grammy made my lunch, I got little sandwiches with no crust, warm tea with sugar and milk, and a cookie, always, a cookie. When Grammy gave me a bath it was done in the kitchen sink, she made sure the water was just right and never once did even a drop of water get in my eyes. I can remember the smells and the feel of those precious nights: the calmingly familiar scent of soap and warm water mixed with a hint of lavender, big scratchy towels that hugged you with sunshine, baby powder with its gentle fragrance, Grammy's caring touch as she rubbed the last bit of powder over my tummy and a boar's hair brush tugging gently over my scalp pulling my wet, baby-fine blond hair into the straight Dutch Boy haircut she had carefully styled for me —baby-fine straight hair with about ten cow-licks. She couldn't do much else with it.

Grammy always put clean pajamas on me. How I loved clean pajamas. To this day I don't like to wear my pajamas for more than one night; of course, they don't smell like the line-dried pajamas of my yesteryear. Then, Grammy would have me kneel at the side of the bed and with folded hands; we would say our prayers together. We would bless everyone in the family first, then the President of our great country, then all the other leaders of the world, and always the starving children of the world, especially the poor starving children of the world. Many a night I went to bed worrying about those poor children. I had never missed a meal and I could not imagine how that could happen. To this day I always remember the children in my prayers. Grammy's hugs were warm, and even though she was a small woman and quite lean, she was cuddly. I am quite sure that by the time she put me in my bed and tucked my covers snugly around me, I was ready to sleep, for all I remember after that was feeling loved.

Yes, indeed, grandparents have a lot to offer, and it is a wise parent who can see this.

I wish you and your family the very best.

Warmest Regards,
Maggie Rose

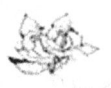

Living in Doubt

Dear Maggie Rose,

My brother and I have not spoken to each other in several years. I am not ready to pick up where we left off, but our mother has become frail and needs more care. This requires more money and our budget is stretched rather thin. My husband wants me to contact my brother and ask him if he can help with the expenses for Mom. I dread making this call and the emotional garbage that I think will follow. I am not sure if I should do this. I really would not call except that I feel I should do this for my husband since he has carried the bulk of the financial burden for my mother's care. Can you shed any light on what I should do and how I should go about this?

Dear Living in Doubt,

I think all of us understand that family relationships can become strained, and working all that through can be exhausting for everyone involved. What we sometimes forget about our siblings is that how our siblings feel about their parent/parents is very different from how they feel toward their siblings. From what you said, I assume your brother

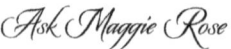
is not current on what is going on with your mother's health or what needs she may have. Since you and your husband have assumed the responsibility for her care, you have assumed the responsibility to communicate about her well-being and her needs to your brother. It comes with the title of caretaker. What he chooses to do, once he has heard what is going on, is his responsibility.

You may learn, and pleasantly so, that your brother would be happy to help with his mother's care in whatever way he can. That is not a promise that sibling issues vanish. They usually don't. The best plan for any dialogue you will have with your brother is to sit down with pen and paper and write out, in vivid detail, every question and every answer you think your brother will have. (What would your questions be if you were in his shoes?). Since your brother won't be current on most of the details, you should be prepared to outline events that have occurred up to this point. Please be prepared to give him some time to mull over your conversation and get back to you with his answer. If it is too difficult for you and your brother to meet and/or talk on your own you could call in a trusted family member or a family counselor to facilitate such a discussion and help you put a plan together.

I hope you have looked into all the resources available to you and your husband as caregivers, and that you have exhausted all avenues available to your mother: private insurance, Medicare, Medicaid. I trust that you know that your local Council on Aging can help you with any needed information or help you find resources that you may have overlooked. You didn't say whether your mother was still in her own home or if she is living with you, and you didn't address how the money would be spent. I am sure your brother will want to know as many details as possible. It is important for you and your husband to know what services are available to you, and I am sure your brother will want to know this kind of information as well. I know there is a program that will pay you for providing care for your mother. In December of 2006, Medicaid funded an Elder Care Program that pays Massachusetts' family caregivers up to $18,000 per year to care for their elders at home. I know that is not near what the care you give is worth, but it is available, and it would be important to know how and where to apply for this type of assistance.

All of us have to be true to ourselves, and sometimes, who we are is not going to mix well with whom someone else is. That is very hurtful when it is family. Just the same, family is family, and I suggest that trying to work together to accomplish something worthy for your mother would give all of you a good deal of comfort in future years. We do not have an indefinite amount of time to resolve all the little hurts (or big ones) that happen in life; sometimes, the healthiest course of action is to forgive the past and move on. Wanting to be forgiven for anything we have done wrong is human. It is just as human to be unable to admit that we might have done something that needs forgiving. Somewhere between those two polarities lies the common denominator that often acts as an equalizer. In the case of you and your brother, the common denominator is the shared love of a parent. It would be wise to try to make that work. It might bring some closure to the past that will help you both have a little more clarity about the real issue: how do you manage caring for your mother?

I wish you and your family the very best.

Warmest Regards,
Maggie Rose

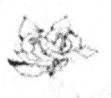

Twenty-Four-Seven Care: Alzheimer's Disease

Dear Maggie Rose,

My dad has early stage Alzheimer's disease and lives at home with my husband and me. Unfortunately, my dad missed the last step coming down the stairs on Sunday morning and fell. He fractured his left humerus bone near his shoulder. It has been difficult for him because the doctors cannot put a cast on the break because of where he broke the bone, but they did put a tight sling on him to hold the arm in place. He is in pain and taking Vicodin for the pain. The Vicodin makes him disconnected and disoriented. I took a few days off from work because he needs constant supervision. He actually keeps forgetting that he fractured his arm, and he is always wondering why his arm hurts so much. This type of behavior happens when the medications set in. In addition, he keeps taking his arm sling off because he says that it is in the way and he cannot use his arm. I have no idea how he gets this done since it is a sling that is braced against his body by going around his neck and his back to keep him from moving his arm. He usually removes it during the night.

I feel this trauma has really set him back and I am worried about it. I am wondering if you know of any resources that I can contact in order to get some "in house" help for my Dad. I am concerned that if I do get in-home help that he will take offense and be abrupt with the help; however, I cannot be here 24/7 because of my job. I will have to call and ask for some personal time. I hope I can take a couple of weeks of leave until his fracture is under control and my Dad can handle more things on his own. I am hopeful that things can return to what they were. I would love to be able to quit my job to be home with him, but these are financially tough times and I feel lucky to have a job right now. I put a call into his doctor to get some advice from him and ask him about other resources. I figured I would reach out to anyone who may know what resources are available. Let me know your thoughts and I am sorry to bother you.

A in Belmont

Dear A,

You are not a bother.

I am sorry about your dad's fall. I am familiar with the type of break he sustained, and it is a difficult break for even the most cooperative of patients to handle. I can also appreciate how complicated this change in his health is for you and your husband and that the confusion he is suffering can only make things more burdensome. I think some in-home help is essential.

I want to thank you for allowing me to share your letter since it does demonstrate the complexity and magnitude of the responsibility that the caregivers assume when they agree to care for a parent with Alzheimer's. The disease makes everything more complicated because the patient cannot understand what is happening to him or her, something that is clearly demonstrated by your father's constant removal of his arm from its brace-sling. He does not remember that he broke his arm, so he cannot understand how important it is to leave the arm in its sling to allow the bone to set—we can all appreciate how difficult it is for the bone to heal if it is constantly disturbed.

I know that you and I have talked privately about the challenges that lie ahead for you and your family. A trauma like the one your family is experiencing right now is a reminder to all of us who bear the responsibility of caretaking that we must also remember to take care of ourselves. Our emotional and financial resources are under a constant strain. It takes a lot of well-organized planning to run a home and manage care for an aging parent. This becomes doubly true with an Alzheimer's patient.

Thank you for taking my advice and contacting the social worker who works at the Senior Center. I trust that some of her suggestions were helpful and that you will continue to reach out to the Council for support.

Here is a web page that I feel is useful for all caretakers: http://www.caring.com/articles/alzheimers-caregivers-need-a-break. As you continue your journey through this difficult time, remember to re-evaluate your plan constantly. Be prepared to be flexible in your thinking and your expectations for your father's future. So much of your dad's progress will be out of your control. Your own mental health and that of your family will rely more on your ability to keep your emotional balance during unpredictable and often frustrating situations. You cannot do that if you are exhausted or frantic. Given these factors, I think in-home help is essential if you are going to try to keep your father at home.

I wish you and your family the best.

Warmest regards,
Maggie Rose

Hello Mother

Today I saw a woman

carrying a vase of red tulips

across the snowy parking lot

in front of the market.

She opened her car door

and placed them

on the front seat of her car.

There was nothing there

to hold the vase

and I wondered

if she planned to drive home

with one hand holding

the vase

and the other

the wheel of her car.

It is probably

what I would do:

take that chance

to bring home the promise of spring.

I got dizzy thinking

about the smell of earth and sun.

I trudged through the snow

to my car

and sat,

with nothing to hold me,

and thought about how much I miss you.

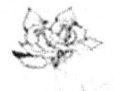

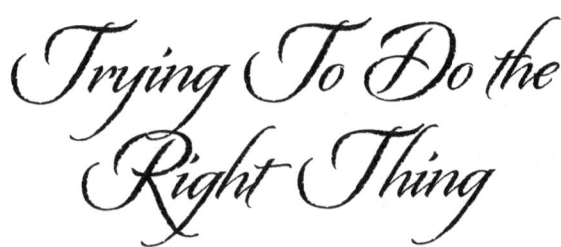

Trying To Do the Right Thing

Dear Maggie Rose,

I need some help deciding what to do next. My mother fell last fall and broke her hip. She is seventy-seven and a widow and I am her only child, so my husband reluctantly agreed that she could come live with us. I expected her to be happy and feel grateful towards my husband and me; instead, she is angry and defensive. The mornings are a nightmare. She needs assistance to dress and undress but yells at me when I am helping her. She makes mean spirited accusations and she is rude. I dread mornings. I am worn out by 9a.m. The rest of my day is a blur. My husband and I are ready to send her packing, but when we mention assisted living, she starts to cry. She wants to stay. I don't want her to go, but things can't continue like this. I am trying to do the right thing.

Name withheld by request.

Dear "Trying to do the right thing",

Taking care of anyone, young or old, is taxing. When it's your parent the emotional drain can overwhelm you. The change in roles is a unique dynamic that requires true finesse and stamina; between mother and daughter, it also requires a lot of extra tenderness. Small indignities have to give way to the larger issue, trust.

Find an opportunity to get your mother's full attention, and then look into her eyes and from your heart tell her how much you love her. Let her know that you are together so you can help her, and that you realize that she doesn't always understand what it is that you are asking of her. Ask her to trust you to do the right things to help make her life better. Talk to her with the same consideration you would want if you were in her shoes. Give her time for your words to sink in. She may need some reassurance that you are not angry with her for all the extra work she has brought into your life. In time, she will let go of her anger and resentment; acceptance and gratitude will follow.

You may want to consider a home health aide to help your mother. This person should be someone you both interview. A home health aide in the mornings seems a viable alternative for your mother's morning routine.

A wonderful support group meets the first Tuesday of every month at 7 p.m. at the Senior Center in Belmont. I think you and your husband would benefit from it. You would meet people who are doing just what you are. A support group is an excellent place to learn some new

"Thrive Skills." Thrive skills is a phrase I like to use for going the extra steps needed to do more than survive.

I wish you and your family the best.

Warmest Regards,
Maggie Rose

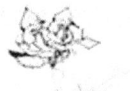

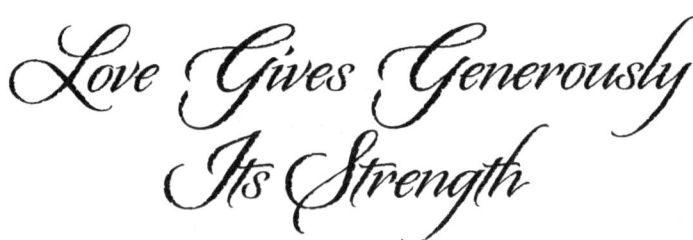

Love Gives Generously Its Strength

Dear Maggie Rose,

I am writing to you because over the holiday something happened to me that speaks to the experience of caregivers and those they care for.

During the holiday, my family was visiting with me from Wisconsin. I went to the grocery store to pick up a few things we needed. I was standing in the dairy section when a man looked up at me while holding some eggnog and said, "I'm getting this for my mother to help put some weight on her."

I laughed at this because I was thinking of my own mother who is trying to keep weight off.

He continued. "She has cancer, and it is hard for her to keep weight on. She likes eggnog and she's even starting to get a little belly from drinking so much of it," he said with a smile. "But she would worry about it, so I don't tell her that."

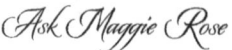

I was touched by how he spoke of her and that he knew her ways and her feelings and the respect he displayed for them as we talked.

I asked him how his mother was doing now, and he confided that it was a tough time of year for them because around the same time last year they lost his dad and his brother in an accident. He quickly went on to explain that his mother weighs ninety pounds soaking wet but that she is the strong one. He furrowed his forehead and explained with quiet tenderness in his voice that she has been the one who has carried him through her illness and the loss of his dad and brother. He paused to gain composure. I was nodding and wiping my eyes.

Then he said, "It's like women have something extra, and it kicks in when we need them."

He paused again. We both had tears in our eyes, the two of us standing in the grocery store talking about something so intimate and important. We wiped our eyes. We went our separate ways, each reminding the other to enjoy the holiday and maybe a bit embarrassed by the emotions we revealed or maybe somewhat surprised that such moments are possible with strangers.

Later that day, I was walking with my brother and he had his three-year-old daughter on his shoulders. We were walking to the coffee shop in my neighborhood. My niece grew restless so my brother put her down, and she raced up the sidewalk. He reminded her to stop at the corner. She turned around to look back at him and then scurried to the edge of the sidewalk and stopped. I watched the two of them, a dad and his daughter, both healthy and strong and enjoying each other. His face showed the joy he felt and how proud of her he was. I told him about my conversation with the stranger. Without words, we both understood.

Wouldn't you agree that there is a small miracle happening when someone with such a frail body can offer such strength to others? Even to the people who are caring for her.

Anonymous in Somerville, MA

Dear Anonymous,

Your letter is beautiful, and it captures the heart of where a woman's strength comes from. Being a caretaker is an act of love, and receiving the care with a loving heart is an act of love. When this loving generosity of heart takes place simultaneously, both are fortified. We are never more loving than when we are vulnerable. Our ability to surrender to our feelings is the greatest strength any of us has as it requires that we trust another human being, and for the frail, that we trust someone with our life.

I wish you and your family the best.

Warmest regards,
Maggie Rose

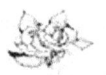

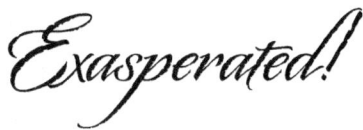

Exasperated!

Dear Maggie Rose,

I am living with a grumpy old man and it is no fun. My husband turned fifty-nine in June of this year, and it's as if the world turned upside down. He is negative about everything that is going on in his life. He worries about everything. He starts the day with a list of complaints and ends it by reassuring himself that he is right to be worried about his job, his boss, the economy, my job, our son, the price of gas, the light bill, how much it will cost to heat the house this winter, his knees pain, his tiredness, my spending too much, paying for our daughter's education, and never being able to retire. Oh my God, the list goes on. It is a serious enough problem that I find myself staying at my mother's house a couple of days a week. Maggie, when I say grumpy, I am being kind. It really borders on abusive. The light bill can set off a twenty-minute temper tantrum followed by two hours of loud reprimands, and the undertone is always that we, the children and I, are the cause of all his woes. It certainly is not healthy. Is he going through a phase? Is this some kind of male menopause? I have heard a few references to such a condition. What do I do about it?

Exasperated

Dear Exasperated,

First, I am not sure what "it" is, so telling you what to do to fix "it" isn't possible for me. Now, for the sake of your marriage, you both need to be clear that you cannot allow this type of dynamic to continue. Abusive behavior is not male menopause, and you are right to get away from it. However, if, up to this point you both have always felt the communication was good and this is a new problem, resolving it will take a little mutual effort. Sometimes, under an emotional strain some bad behaviors will surface. You do need to hold your husband accountable for his behavior. Let him know you feel he is being verbally abusive. Be sure he is clear that his tone and negativity are the reasons that you are going to your mothers. Offer him some other ways to talk to you; he may have forgotten how to express unpleasant feelings.

I am sure you know that I am a great proponent of therapy, and, at the very least, a few healthy sessions with a good marriage counselor will help. Your husband may feel there are a few things he would rather talk over in private. That would be fine too.

Fifty-nine is not old, so when you say "grumpy old man" it does make me think that on some level his behavior does have something to do with age or aging. It is possible that for your husband turning fifty-nine had significance tied to something from his past or some hallmark or accomplishment he feels he has not reached and should have. He may feel frightened that he is not going to meet some preconceived ideal. This may be a good time to open a dialogue about expectations versus reality. Talk to him about what you feel is important in your life together, and remind him of all the things that you are pleased with. Then point out to him the importance of a grateful heart. It is almost impossible to be unhappy when you are thinking about all of the things in your life that are pleasing to you.

We all run hot and cold at different times in our lives. It is not uncommon for anyone, man or woman, to find reaching a certain age unsettling. (That is why I am still thirty-nine.) I love the phrase, "Growing old is not for sissies." It is not!

It takes courage to face the troubles that come with letting go of our youth and moving toward fewer sunsets, but it is exactly because there are fewer sunsets ahead of us that we should embrace them wholeheartedly. Negativity is a drain on everyone. Remind your husband that it is a foolish man who wastes the rewards of his life's work by bemoaning the efforts it took to accomplish them or the cost of maintaining them. Nagging, complaining, whining, and temper tantrums are all forms of childish behaviors. When a grown man uses those kinds of behaviors to control or intimidate his wife and family, what he does is show them—and sadly so—that he undervalues them or, even worse, that he holds them in contempt. What a nasty little boomerang that is for a baby boomer to be throwing around.

I wish you and your family the best.

Warmest regards,
Maggie Rose

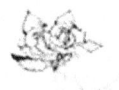

Concerned Grandson

Dear Maggie Rose,

I am the grandson of a veteran and the son of a baby boomer who both live in Belmont. Presently, Congress has a bill before it to vote on called H.R.3200, the Affordable Health Choices Act, which, as I understand it, has little to do with making health care affordable or enacting health care reform. This bill proposes to eliminate up to fifty billion dollars in funding to nursing home care for seniors who will be expecting and needing access to care under their Medicare Part A benefit. Passage of this bill, as it stands, will eliminate essential funding for nursing homes that are paid by the Part A benefit of Medicare for up to a one-hundred-day stay.

This benefit is most often used for post acute hospital stays for rehabilitation back to home. This is not about long-term nursing home care but about the rehabilitation that is needed for infirm patients after things like heart surgery, a hip fracture, hip or knee replacement surgery, and other significant medical conditions that require a rehabilitation period for the patient to recuperate and then return home. This care, once provided in hospitals, is now provided in short-term nursing facilities, which is the more cost effective way to handle this type of care.

It does not make sense to cut funding to those who will be providing the care for a population that will be increasing demand for care. As the baby boomer generation ages, there will be a greater demand for this service and costs will naturally continue to increase. If Congress votes to remove funding for this service at this time, it will lead to drastic cuts and limited access for those seeking rehabilitation services in the near future. I do not believe many seniors are aware of the intended cuts to Part A benefits, and I wanted to bring it to your attention. The proposed focus is to bring the patients, without rehabilitation, back into their homes where their families can then assume the management of the "patients'" rehabilitation needs.

I strongly urge people to write their congressional representatives and express how they feel about cuts to skilled nursing facilities.

Thank you for listening,

R. P., a concerned grandson

Dear R. P.,

Thank you for bringing this to my attention. As a member of the baby boomer generation and the primary caretaker for my mother during her many bouts with short-term rehabilitation, I am very sensitive to the need for this service. If you read my last column, you know that rehabilitation is often the first stop for a loved one on their journey home after a significant hospital stay. Without that interim step, many of our loved ones would be sent home unable to resume their normal adult daily living tasks: grooming, bathing, climbing stairs, reaching, bending, cooking, reading, and even speaking. I can appreciate your concern that these services, now provided by benefits included in Medicare Part A, might be lost.

As we age, the human body does not recover as quickly as it did in youth. Three days in bed due to a serious illness is often enough that an elderly patient will require physical therapy in order to return safely home. After heart surgery or a stroke, it is mandatory that a patient receive rehabilitation. Rehabilitation after knee or hip surgery is an assumed part of the process of recovery. It is frightening how quickly reform can turn into refuse. I think we all have to make a serious effort to educate ourselves in regards to this complicated subject and keep our representatives informed. We do need to demand clarity on the details of what *reform* would mean for all involved, so we can then weigh the gains and the losses in an effort to reach an equitable and realistic solution to a monumental issue.

I am not making any commentary about HR3200 either pro or con. I do agree with you that my readers would be interested in knowing what is being proposed and making their own choice about how to respond. I would like to provide a web site: www.Thomas.loc.gov. You can search the bill by name: HR 3200, once that comes on, there is a hyperlink to areas of the bill that have to do with long-term care, homecare and caregiver issues. Once you get there, you can see all the amendments related to those issues. Most of them concern having nursing homes more accountable (as if they weren't already), organizing them somewhat differently, and channeling nursing home dollars to homecare—something we're already doing in Massachusetts.

I wish you and your family the best.

Warmest regards,
Maggie Rose

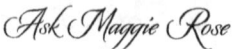

A Soldier's Lament

Blood trumpeted the tears fall;

I heard the thunderous explosion;

I saw the pieces of my brothers spewed

upon a crusted land of sand;

I heard the ululations of

their wounded women;

strange lament for a soldier.

Eyeless, the world watches;

I am judged by my presence here;

We cannot leave enough of ourselves:

The bits and pieces of our bodies,

The duty paid to remain;

strange lament for a soldier.

I had a mother once.

She smiled bravely when I died;

She knew it was better

than the wound still left:

The challenge of freedom

without this war;

strange lament for a soldier.

Maggie Rose

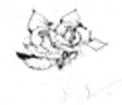

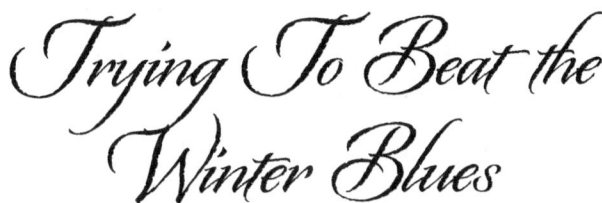

Trying To Beat the Winter Blues

Dear Maggie Rose,

I've been taking care of my increasingly sick, elderly mother, and my grown children are out of state dealing with some serious family issues of their own. It is depressing to think of how I wish things would be as things are so overwhelming to me right now. I don't really want to give up but I don't see any way to make the next several weeks of winter better especially over the upcoming holidays. What can I do to beat the winter blues?

Trying To Beat The Winter Blues.

Dear "Trying To Beat The Winter Blues,"

It was your word choice, "It is depressing to think about how I wish things would be," that I want most to respond to because that little phrase is a peek into thinking that can start the blues. I guess my response is that we should begin to change how we think when we first realize that we are in a slump. It is natural, especially during the holidays, when winter first starts to settle in that we feel some stress. There is enough holiday hype out there, and all of it is designed to focus our attention on a Wall Street version of what a perfect holiday should be (I think we can pick it up at a local retail store), that it is easy to start thinking about what is lacking from our lives. However, in the real world, mother is failing and children are dealing with serious family issues. So when we are dealing with real issues, where we focus our thoughts might be the single most important thing we can do for ourselves.

Dwelling on how we wish things were is similar to sitting on the fence when you have a decision to make. We waste our energy imagining what things might be like. When we embrace how things are, we can spend that same energy doing things that make us happy. Therefore, the first thing you can do to make for a more joyous holiday season is make a decision to accept how things are. Now you are ready to allow some joy into your heart. One of the hardest lessons in life is to learn that you can be unhappy about one set of circumstances and still find happiness in other interest, but self-obsession is a bottomless pit.

Make something by hand for your mother. Make it about her and present it to her with a big bow and a tender heart. It will give you memories that will last for many years. Do something generous for a children's organization. Plan a trip with your children for a future year. Ask them to pick from two or three different destinations. Make it a family gift. Make a new friend. Cook something from another part of the world. Go online and learn about the country and the food. Buy a gift for every resident in a local long-term nursing facility. Spend a day handing out your gifts, or do the same at a group home for adolescents.

The key thing is to stop thinking about you. In case you haven't noticed, you are a bit depressing; I do hope your humor is intact enough that you can laugh with me on that.

The main thing is to get involved. You need to be proactive. You are Saint Nick. The holiday is up to you. If anything is going to happen at your house, or not happen, it will be because of you. Furthermore, that is true for the rest of the year too.

I wish you and your family the best.

Warmest regards,
Maggie Rose

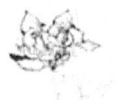

Barking up the Wrong Tree

Dear Maggie Rose,

My mother is seventy-three. She has been living with us since my father died last summer in June. She recently had a heart attack. She is recovering well, but I can tell she is depressed. I am worried about her, and I want to do something to help her. I noticed she seems very fond of our neighbors' dogs, and I have heard that a pet can be a big help for someone with depression. I have hinted that she should get a dog but she will always brush it off with a comment like, "It's too much work," or "It would just be one more thing to do around here."

She and my dad had a terrier named Sparky for years. I know she loved the dog; he practically ran the house. She even prepared his dinner at the same time she and dad ate so they could all eat together. Should I go ahead and get one for her or am I barking up the wrong tree?

Dear Barking Up The Wrong Tree,

I am happy to hear your that mother is doing well. You are lucky to have each other. It is good that you are asking before you jump right in

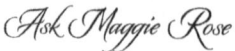

and bring a dog home. I am not saying no—that is how my mother used to put me on hold. I am saying let us think about all of the questions you are really bringing up. Your mother lost her husband, she moved out of her own home and into yours, and she had a major illness, all in the span of ten months. There are many details left out, but almost any scenario I can think of would put anyone into a tailspin. I hope your mother isn't depressed. I think she may be grieving, and, honestly, maybe you are too. The normal grieving process takes time. I think your mother needs time to be sad. I think I understand how her sadness makes you feel. Obviously, you love her and don't want her to suffer. My friend, we cannot fix everything. Sometimes the best thing you can do is give someone the emotional space to go through the paces that life requires. Be there for each other and spend some of that together time talking about Sparky. It sounds like there were plenty of happy memories for your mother during Sparky's reign. Fond memories heal the heart in more ways than you can count.

I love dogs. If it turns out that at some point down the road you and your mother do decide together to get a dog, I can speak with some authority when I say that dogs and pets in general, but dogs especially, are a healthy addition to most peoples' lives.

There are numerous studies—way too many to try and mention—that suggest that older citizens experience tremendous benefits from being around or owning pets. I remember reading something very recently that suggested that heart attack patients who owned pets often were ten times more likely to survive beyond the first year than non-owners were. I can't remember the source but I believe it anyway.

The United States Humane Society points out a number of benefits to pet ownership: "Pets provide companionship and give people someone to care for. Because they provide a focus of conversation and activity, pets help people to be more sociable. Pets comfort people with touch and stimulate exercise."

There are many reasons to get a dog and your mother would, most likely, benefit from the companionship of a friendly dog. The dog, however, will not stop grief. Take your time with this decision. I feel fairly certain that with love and patience your mother and you will start to enjoy more lighthearted days. Days that will be made all the sweeter because of the time you have spent healing together. If puppy loves were to be a part of your lives, well then, wouldn't you be lucky?

I wish you and your family the best.

Warmest regards,
Maggie Rose

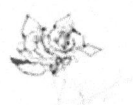

A Devoted Nurse's Aide

Dear Maggie Rose,

Since I first came to this country, I have worked in the same nursing home in Arlington. During that time, I have watched how people in this country treat their parents. They send them to a nursing home and then visit twice a year. Some never visit. Some visit and never talk with the parent. In my country, we respect our elders and we take care of them. I often feel disgusted by the lack of love I have witnessed. I have even seen children come in and demand that a parent be placed into hospice care because they think the parent is taking too long to die because we give them such good care. I hope that this Father's Day more people will think about their fathers and give them the attention they deserve.

A Devoted Nurse's Aide

Dear Devoted,

First, let me thank you for the job you do.

While I admit that nursing homes aren't usually pleasant places to visit, I think you are being judgmental. I, too, worked in a nursing facility,

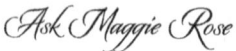

and I made the same judgment call that you have. Over the years, I have picked up some wisdom that allows me to see things differently.

I don't know what country you come from, but *respect* isn't what visiting a parent in a nursing home is about. You visit out of love or a sense of duty sometimes both. You visit to share some news or watch a game together. You visit because you can. Not everyone can.

As parents, we raise our children, ultimately, to be independent and self-sufficient. Most modern families have relatives living in many different and often distant parts of the county and even the world. Every person with whom I have ever talked to about retirement wanted to remain independent. The decision to go to a nursing facility is never easy, but the reason for the decision is always some event or condition that caused a loved one to need a different level of care. The results are the burdens that the family shares.

Just as you left your country to come to America, many young Americans left their home state to find jobs that could better their lives. Most families have two working parents and children in school or college. They have full, active lives. This is what their parents wanted for them. Rarely do circumstances make opportunities for children to bring the comfort and care to their parents that they might wish they could. I am sure there is a lot of guilt and pain around that issue. I wouldn't sit in judgment of that.

I understand why someone who works as an aide may make the unfortunate leap that you have made about hospice care. I have the greatest respect for all hospice workers. The decision to choose hospice care is often a very difficult but, ultimately, a loving act on the part of the family. Hospice isn't just for cancer patients; it is for palliative care when a patient isn't expected to live longer than six months.

Do what you do with a happy heart and forget about what you think should be. I have seen nurse's aides who have three and four children at home work back-to-back seventy-hour workweeks. There are folks who might sit in judgment of that. I won't.

I wish you and your family the best.

Warmest regards,
Maggie Rose

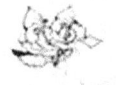

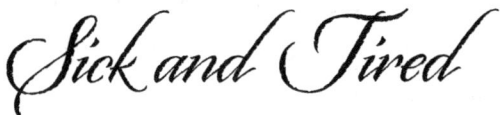

Sick and Tired

Dear Maggie Rose,

I'm exhausted. I am tired of the weather. I am tired of all the extra clothes. I am tired of waiting for the weather to change. I am just plain tired. I am too tired to even think. I am not sick; I am just sick and tired. How can I "get away" without spending a fortune and without leaving my responsibilities?

Tired In Belmont.

Dear Tired In Belmont,

Here is a list of my top ten rejuvenators. Each one of them can fit neatly into even the most hectic of schedules. They all cost less than one hundred dollars. They work wonders for me so I hope they work for you.

Maggie Rose's Top Ten Stress Relievers

1. Buy a small aquarium. You can order many on line. The cost is reasonable. You will be surprised at the calming effect that setting up a small aquarium can have.

2. Have a qualified massage therapist come to your home and give you a full hour of skilled deep tissue massage. Be sure to let your therapist know the massage is for relaxation. If you're not comfortable with someone coming to your home, go to his or her office for the massage.

3. Throw everyone out of the house for two hours. Have ready some scented candles, bath salts, thick luxurious towels, a glass of sherry or wine, a great album, and a tub full of hot water. Put the bath salts in the tub of water, sip your sherry, make sure the towels are close at hand, start the music, light the candles, sip your sherry again, get in the tub, adjust the water temperature according to your needs, and soak in the tub. After your bath take a nap. You will sleep like a baby and wake up refreshed. I promise.

4. Get a pedicure. I am not recommending the manicure since most men aren't interested in one and I have found that many women are impatient while trying to sit still long enough to let their nails dry properly, hardly the effect we are going for. The pedicure, however, seems to have the opposite effect. Go to a salon that has a massage therapy chair. Ladies, shave your legs the day before you go, not on the day you go. I think it is a little healthier that way. Bring sandals to wear home.

5. Learn some Zen meditation. There are few things more relaxing than clearing the mind. You can go online and find a sampling of meditation centers. Pick one that sounds like fun to you and go.

6. Buy a gift for a dear friend and invite her or him over for a cup of tea. Have the present gift wrapped or wrap it yourself, but go all out. Give it as an unbirthday present. The joy the two of you will share will make you smile for days. You will forget you are tired.

7. Get your hair washed and set or washed and blow-dried. Don't make any changes; don't do it for any reason except that you can. Make sure you tell your stylist that you are doing it just for fun. I wouldn't try this on a weekend unless you plan ahead with the salon or scheduling might be a problem.

8. Buy yourself some new bedroom slippers and stay in your pajamas all weekend. Tell your family you're taking a few sick days at home. Do only what you feel like doing, nothing else. Order all your meals delivered or don't eat anything at all, whichever is easiest for you. Always drink plenty of water. It's great for the skin and has a true detoxifying effect.

9. Invite some friends over to play a board game. Play as if you are children. Serve popcorn and soft drinks. Take some time to enjoy the playfulness of your youth. I think this is a blast and it is amazing how many new things you will find to like about your playmates.

10. Get out of the house. Go to a movie. See a show. You need to change the scenery. The hardest part of this is getting out the door. Go alone or go with a friend or a family member, but go. Even a trip to Starbucks can make the world go away for a while. Curl up on one of their big overstuffed chairs with a nice cup of cappuccino and do some people watching. It works!

I wish you and your family the best.

Warmest regards,
Maggie Rose

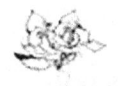

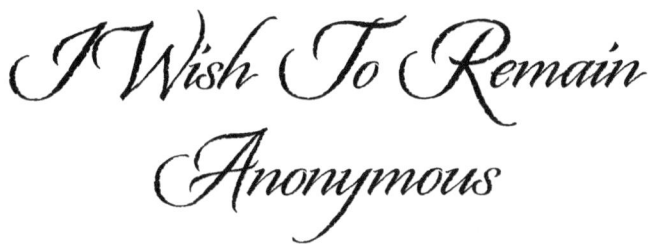

I Wish To Remain Anonymous

Dear Maggie Rose,

My husband and I will have been married fifty years this June. We have loved each other through the good times and the bad times. When we got married we had nothing but our love and each other. Fifty years later, we still have our love and each other, and we have four children, eight grandchildren, and a dog. We own two homes; one is a nice property at the shore, and the other is here in suburban Boston. Marriage is never easy, but, looking back, ours was as easy as they come. It has been a good life with many good times and very little sadness. Unfortunately, I am at the end of my life. I have been diagnosed with terminal cancer.

I haven't kept many secrets from my husband, but I have been able to keep this from him. I can't bear to bring this hurt to him or the children. I am worried about how he will handle things when I am gone; I have always been his rock and I know this. Mostly, I am just sad. My husband and I built our life together; we were husband and wife first, then mother and father, and we were always a family. Our children have planned a nice gathering for our fiftieth anniversary. I might tell my husband about my health issues some time after the party. Can you believe this is the one thing I do not know how to tell him? I am not sure I want to. Can you advise me?

Sincerely,
I wish to remain anonymous.

Dear Anonymous,

Yes, I believe you. It is difficult to face the news of our own impending death, and sharing that news with a loved one can be equally difficult and make it even more real. I am sorry for your sad news. I think that facing one's own death can be terrifying, and doing that alone is simply too much. You need to confide in someone about your own fears for yourself and so that you don't project your wish that it not be so on to others. None of us is getting out of this life alive. We all know this, yet the news of our own mortality is always shocking. If you are too frightened, it will only convey to your husband and loved ones that your impending death is too much for any one of you to bear. Though it may well feel that way to you now, if you could find some person who could share the "rock" role when you do tell your husband, it may feel less like you are leaving him stranded with the news. This person could help hold—embrace you both as a couple and a family—you through the discussions and ease some of the emotional burden. Your husband may be too fragile to handle this without the support of someone else, or you may find that he will be able to be your rock for this. Whatever may happen, that extra person could give both you and your husband some much-needed support. I am sure you know him best and will choose the most comforting path for both of you.

Hospice care is available to anyone whose doctor gives him or her a prognosis of six months or less, but, to reassure you, many, many people live longer than their prognoses. The therapeutic aspects of hospice stays seem to help some people live longer. You have been brave enough to confront the fact that you are dying. That is good because denial is an unfortunate block towards getting the right kind of support and help. In a sense, right now your whole family needs to be held. Hospice care is a way the whole family could be "held."

You probably remember a time—I certainly do— when cancer was a dirty word. If someone in your household died from cancer, people would lie and say that their loved one died from a heart attack or some other more acceptable form of death. How absurd! I hope you don't have any of that old kind of thinking holding you back from doing what you know you must. You must say goodbye to your love, your friend, your husband, father of your children, master of your dog, and coconspirator in your life. Together you can prepare your children and say goodbye to the many others in your life. You and your husband built this life together; you will finish it together, even if you have to leave first. No matter what, life is a day-by-day event. None of us knows when some unforeseen event might change life as we know it today. There is a reason you haven't kept many secrets from your husband. Secrets don't work well in a marriage.

I know there are actual steps involved in the process of accepting the kind of news you have received. I think denial and avoidance are among the first of those steps. I can also appreciate your desire to protect someone you love. I am sure, after fifty years of marriage, you have learned that love doubles joy and divides sorrow. Are you going to deny your husband the chance to be your rock, if, in fact, he is able to do this for you? Every day that you keep this from him, you may be shortchanging both of you and wasting precious time that you could be spending going through this together. Where do you find the comfort you need? When you are gone, how will your husband find comfort if you leave him believing two things: you could not turn to him for comfort, and you could not trust him to take care of you?

There are all kinds of guidelines for dealing with cancer. Get the information out in front of your husband and follow your hearts for dealing with the rest. Your two hearts have guided you through almost 50 years of happiness together; they can make this last journey together. Here are a few steps for you both. I found them listed under Wellness Junction (www.wellnessjunction.com/athome/disease_prevention/coping.htm), a website I turn to for information from time to time:

"1. **Be open with your fears and anxieties about the disease** — It is common the patient and the caregiver are frightened by a cancer diagnosis. That is why it is important for both of you to sit down and discuss your fears and concerns up front...

"2. **Assist in treatment decisions** — It is important the supporting caregiver and the patient face the difficult decisions about diagnosis and treatment together. If possible, both should attend the meetings with the doctor where treatment decisions will be discussed. It may help to decrease your anxieties...

"3. **Provide a comfortable environment for the cancer patient** — By paying attention to the details of comfort for your loved one, you will help them have to deal with one less item on their emotional plate.

"4. **Maintain a balance for yourself** — It is important you and the person you care for continue to take time for the usual day-to-day activities. This will help you feel less overwhelmed and keep a healthy life balance.

"5. **Don't be afraid to seek the support of others** — People don't need to face cancer by themselves. Seek the support of other family members and friends, other cancer patients, religious help, cancer support groups, doctors, and mental health professionals.

"'By following these steps and facing cancer together it can strengthen everything that is good in a relationship ... Providing a supportive environment helps the patient's and family's ability to deal with the crisis, promotes mutual support, and helps to sustain relationships.'

For more information, visit: www.nfcr.org."

I admire your courage, and I understand your thinking; however, you are not thinking clearly. Your wonderful marriage can support both of you through this if you honor your husband and your love with the same honesty that you have enjoyed for fifty years. I wish I could say or do something more for you that might make the time ahead easier. Please know I will keep you in my thoughts and prayers, and I am sure that many of my readers will as well. I hope the two of you and your family enjoy, to the fullest, your fiftieth anniversary celebration.

I wish you and your family the best.

Warmest regards,
Maggie Rose

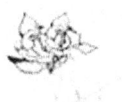

A Reader In Need

Dear Maggie Rose,

Hi,

Could you send me the article you wrote in the *Belmont-Citizen Herald* the week of September 4? It was about caregivers making sure that they take care of themselves. I *need* that article!

What spoke to me most eloquently was the part about not letting yourself become one of the living dead. It read, "Stay happy about what is good in your life and take pride and comfort in the loving care you do give your mother, but do remember to take care of yourself."

I think that I have been one of the living dead and have been quite depressed over the years. It is not just caring for an aged parent; what has been even more difficult in my life has been dealing with a difficult sibling: a brother who has major issues and is passive-aggressive and critical.

I need to collaborate with him for the sake of my mother's care. The stress of that alliance is something that has been, and continues to be, extremely difficult for me to do.

A Reader In Need

Dear Reader In Need,

The first thing you need is a big hug. I don't know how hard it has been for you, but I do get a sense of how worn out you are by the struggle to keep your brother involved.

You feel you need his help; do you really need his help? The question I am asking is if you can replace the care he provides your mom—I know that means some time off for you—with people who provide qualified, private-pay help? If you can minimize your dependence on him for assistance, you can remove the emotional traps that a passive-aggressive and critical sibling brings to an already demanding and draining situation. Your mental health is worth whatever it may cost. Hopefully, your mother will be able to pay for this aid. You cannot fix your brother, but you can do something about how much interaction you subject yourself to.

We have a great caregivers support group which meets at the Beech Street Center, the first Tuesday of every month at seven in the evening. Everything you share will be kept confidential. It is a small group made up of couples and singles, daughters, sons, and the Director of the Council on Aging, Nava Niv-Vogel, facilitates it. I could not do what I do for my mother without the guidance I receive there.

Also, we have a *Caregiver's Bill of Rights* that we hand out at the meeting to the new people. I want to share it with you here because I think it will help you. The intention is to have it act as a written reminder of how delicate the ties that bind us to duty, honor, and love really are. We must claim for ourselves all the dignity we give to our loved ones while we care for them. Every unselfish, kind, and loving thing we do for them, we must do for ourselves. To do otherwise is to be a hypocrite in all that we profess to hold sacred as a caregiver. To truly value life, we must start with our own.

I wish you and your family the best.

Warmest regards,
Maggie Rose

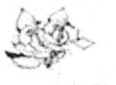

A Caregiver's Bill of Rights

I have the right:

1. To take care of myself. This is not an act of selfishness. It will give me the capability of taking better care of my loved one.

2. To seek help from others even though my loved one may object. I recognize the limits of my own endurance and strength.

3. To maintain facets of my own life that do not include the person I care for, just as I would if he or she were healthy. I know that I do everything that I reasonably can for this person, and I have the right to do some things just for myself.

4. To get angry, be depressed and express other difficult feelings occasionally.

5. To reject any attempt by my loved one (either conscious or unconscious) to manipulate me through guilt, anger or depression.

6. To receive consideration, affection, forgiveness, and acceptance for what I do from my loved one as long as I offer these qualities in return.

7. To take pride in what I am accomplishing and to applaud the courage it has sometimes taken to meet the needs of my loved one.

8. To protect my individuality and my right to make a life for myself which will sustain me in the time when my loved one no longer needs my full time help.

9. To accept nothing less than respect from my siblings and extended family who share in the love of my loved one. They may not know or understand all that I do for my loved one, but because I do, I will not accept behavior that is disrespectful of me. I will show the same respectful behavior toward them.

10. To expect and demand that as new strides are made in finding resources to aid physically and mentally impaired older persons in our county, similar strides will be made toward aiding and supporting caregivers.

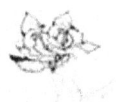

Departed

A kiss upon thy still cold lips,

No feeling in this gentleness,

Silken hair

And tenderness,

My soul

Mate.

Gone,

I reach for you, Feel emptiness

Places in me I know exist.

You are lost to my embrace,

Yet I hold you,

Can I give my life for yours,

My life

Mate?

Yearning,

Tearing,

At my core,

For there was yet much more:

To give, to do, to say,

His snarled, choking, gasping, grip,

Took hold of life,

Then you left.

I watched,

In trance-like drift:

He dealt his final blow,

You succumbed,

Closed not your eyes

To look at me

Did you see that?

They ask of me,

I can only weep.

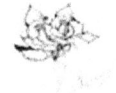

Maggie Rose lives in Belmont, Massachusetts with her husband, her teenage grandson, and her stepdad. She is active in the community and is a caregiver for her dad in their home in Belmont. The Belmont Council on Aging endorses her column. You can reach Maggie Rose at maggiero8@verizon.net or send your mail to Ask Maggie Rose, 266 Beech Street, Belmont, MA 02478.

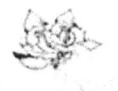

www.ingramcontent.com/pod-product-compliance
Lightning Source LLC
Chambersburg PA
CBHW060638290526
45793CB00001B/305